87 Post Chemotherapy Juice and Meal Recipes:

Get Stronger and Feel More Vitality with These Nutrient Rich Ingredients

By

Joe Correa CSN

COPYRIGHT

This publication is designed to provide accurate and authoritative information in regard to the subject matter covered. It is sold with the understanding that neither the author nor the publisher is engaged in rendering medical advice. If medical advice or assistance is needed, consult with a doctor. This book is considered a guide and should not be used in any way detrimental to your health. Consult with a physician before starting this nutritional plan to make sure it's right for you.

ACKNOWLEDGEMENTS

This book is dedicated to my friends and family that have had mild or serious illnesses so that you may find a solution and make the necessary changes in your life.

87 Post Chemotherapy Juice and Meal Recipes:

Get Stronger and Feel More Vitality with These Nutrient Rich Ingredients

By

Joe Correa CSN

CONTENTS

ABOUT THE AUTHOR

After years of Research, I honestly believe in the positive effects that proper nutrition can have over the body and mind. My knowledge and experience has helped me live healthier throughout the years and which I have shared with family and friends. The more you know about eating and drinking healthier, the sooner you will want to change your life and eating habits.

Nutrition is a key part in the process of being healthy and living longer so get started today. The first step is the most important and the most significant.

INTRODUCTION

87 Post Chemotherapy Juice and Meal Recipes: Get Stronger and Feel More Vitality with These Nutrient Rich Ingredients

By Joe Correa CSN

Chemotherapy can be exhausting and recovering should be your number 1 priority. After you've finished with chemotherapy, there is one important issue that still remains in your life: how to improve your overall health in the best possible way and enjoy the life ahead of you.

No matter what your age and gender, the key to a healthier life lies in a few basic things: a balanced, diet, exercise, and maintaining a healthy body weight. But, the first and most important thing is a balanced diet. That's the base for a strong recovery after you have dealt with your condition.

In order to help you maintain a balanced diet rich in vitamins, proteins, fibers, etc., I have created a collection of meal and juice recipes that will give you a quick and easy solution for eating healthy during the post-chemotherapy period.

Every individual has different symptoms after the treatment, but all of them have one thing in common, a delicate organism that needs some fast recovery.

The recipes in this book were created by following a simple rule: the more nutrients, the better. That is what your body needs at this moment, and that is what I want to give you. Try as many of the recipes as possible to see which ones you enjoy the most.

87 POST CHEMOTHERAPY JUICE AND MEAL RECIPES: GET STRONGER AND FEEL MORE VITALITY WITH THESE NUTRIENT RICH INGREDIENTS

MEALS

1.   Mountain Sandwiches

Ingredients:

1 head of Iceberg lettuce

1 medium-sized tomato, sliced

6 slices of buckwheat bread

For cream:

1 tbsp of almonds

2 tbsp of skim milk

½ cup of goat's cheese, crumbled

2 tbsp of walnuts

¼ tbsp of balsamic vinegar

½ tsp of black pepper, ground

½ tsp of salt

1 tsp of chia seeds

Preparation:

Combine almonds, walnuts, pepper, and salt in a food processor. Add milk, vinegar, and cheese. Blend until you get a smooth creamy mixture. Transfer to a mixing bowl and stir in one teaspoon of chia seeds. Set aside.

Line one leaf of lettuce and 1-2 slices of tomato onto bread slice. Spread the cream mixture equally over the slice, and cover with another lettuce leaf and bread slice.

Nutrition information per serving: Kcal: 143, Protein: 10.4g, Carbs: 21.4g, Fats: 12.4g

2.   Peppers in Cream

Ingredients:

1 cup of Feta cheese, crumbled

1 medium-sized bell pepper, cut into bite-sized pieces

1 tbsp of extra virgin olive oil

2 free-range eggs

½ tsp of salt

½ tsp of ginger

Preparation:

First, boil the eggs. Gently place two eggs in a pot of boiling water. Cook for 10 minutes. Rinse and drain. Cool for a while and peel. You can add one teaspoon of baking soda in a boiling water. This will make the peeling process much easier. Cut the eggs into bite-sized pieces and transfer to a food processor.

Add salt, ginger, and cheese. Blend for 30 seconds or until smooth. Transfer the mixture to a serving bowl.

Add chopped pepper and stir well. Refrigerate for about 30 minutes before serving.

Nutrition information per serving: Kcal: 143, Protein: 10.4g, Carbs: 21.4g, Fats: 12.4g

3.   Winter Frost

Ingredients

1 cup of Greek yogurt

1 tsp of coconut flour

1 small peach, halved and pit removed

1 tsp of mint, ground

1 tbsp of honey

1 tsp of red apple zest

½ tsp of vanilla extract

Preparation:

Combine all ingredients in a food processor except apple zest, in a food processor. Blend until smooth and transfer to the serving glasses.

Sprinkle the top with coconut flour and apple zest.

Refrigerate at least one hour before serving.

Nutrition information **per serving:** Kcal: 172, Protein: 12.3g, Carbs: 29.5g, Fats: 18.4g

4. Wild Blueberry Parfait

Ingredients:

½ cup of fresh wild blueberries

2 tbsp of blueberry extract

1 cup of milk

2 tbsp of milk cream

1 large egg

2 egg whites

1 tbsp of honey

Preparation:

Gently warm the milk in a large pot over a medium-low temperature. Spoon in the cream and continue to stir constantly. You don't want it to boil! Remove from the heat and set aside to cool for a while.

Add the egg, egg whites, honey, and fresh blueberries. Give it a final stir and refrigerate overnight or at least 3-4 hours before serving.

Nutrition information per serving: Kcal: 272, Protein: 12.4g, Carbs: 62.4g, Fats: 18.4g

5.   Cooked Sea Brass with Horseradish Sauce

Ingredients:

2 lb of Sea Brass, boneless

1 medium-sized onion, chopped

2 oz of cherry tomatoes, halved

½ cup of celery, chopped

2 tbsp of fresh parsley, finely chopped

1 medium-sized carrot, sliced

2 tbsp of olive oil

2 garlic cloves, chopped

2 tbsp of lemon juice

1 tsp of vegetable seasoning mix

1 tsp of black pepper, ground

1 tsp of salt

Water

For sauce:

1 oz of prepared horseradish

¼ cup of sour cream

1 ts of salt

1 tbsp of capers

Preparation:

Place the fish and vegetables into the large pot and pour over water until it covers all ingredients. Add lemon juice, pepper, olive oil, and cover with a lid. Cook for about 30 minutes on low heat. Remove from the heat and set aside to cool.

Meanwhile, combine all sauce ingredients in a mixing bowl. Stir well to combine.

Drain the fish and vegetables and transfer to the serving plate. Drizzle some sauce over the fish and vegetables.

You can serve some lemon slices for extra flavor.

Enjoy!

Nutrition information per serving: Kcal: 332, Protein: 32.1g, Carbs: 10.3g, Fats: 13.4g

6.   Quinoa Prunes Bars

Ingredients:

4 tbsp of quinoa, pre-cooked

2 medium-sized bananas, sliced

1 cup of oatmeal

1 free-range egg

1 tsp of cinnamon

1 tsp of flaxseed

½ cup of prunes, finely chopped

1 tbsp of almonds, finely chopped

¼ tbsp of salt

1 tbsp of vegetable oil

Preparation:

Preheat the oven to 400°F.

Combine banana and egg into mixing bowl. Using a fork, whisk well to combine. Set aside.

Take a large mixing bowl and combine all ingredients. Add cooked quinoa and mashed banana-egg mixture. Give it a final stir and transfer to a baking sheet.

Bake for about 25 minutes, or until nicely golden brown. Remove from the oven and set aside to cool for a while.

Cut into equal pieces and serve with milk, but it is, however, optional.

Nutrition information per serving: Kcal: 152, Protein: 9.9g, Carbs: 23.5g, Fats: 4.8g

7.   Potato Bean Salad

Ingredients:

3 cups of green beans, pre-cooked

2 medium-sized potatoes, peeled, cubed and pre-cooked

2 tbsp of capers

2 large eggs, pre-cooked, peeled and sliced into wedges

1 tbsp of fresh parsley, finely chopped

For dressing:

½ cup of sour cream, low-fat

1 tsp of Dijon mustard

1 tbsp of lemon juice

½ tsp of balsamic vinegar

½ tsp of black pepper, ground

Preparation:

Combine all dressing ingredients in a mixing bowl. Stir well to combine and set aside.

Combine beans, capers and potato cubes into a large serving bowl. Top with egg wedges and drizzle with dressing to taste.

For some extra taste, sprinkle with fresh parsley, and serve.

Enjoy!

Nutrition information per serving: Kcal: 252, Protein: 8.7g, Carbs: 32.5g, Fats: 10.8g

8.   Siberian Eggs

Ingredients:

6 free-range eggs

½ cup of Circassian cheese, crumbled

½ cup of heavy cream

1 tbsp of fresh parsley, finely chopped

1 tbsp of honey

Preparation:

Place two eggs in a pot of boiling water and cook for about 10 minutes. Rinse and drain. Cool for a while and set aside.

Meanwhile, combine cheese, parsley, and heavy cream in a large mixing bowl. Now, peel and cut the eggs into bite-sized pieces and transfer to the creamy mixture.

Top with honey and refrigerate for 20 minutes before serving.

Nutrition information per serving: Kcal: 208, Protein: 13.5g, Carbs: 10.7g, Fats: 13.6g

9.   Creamed Greens

Ingredients:

6 oz of kale, chopped

6 oz of spinach, chopped

4 oz of Brussel sprouts, halved

2 cups of vegetable broth

½ tsp of black pepper, ground

For cream:

2 tbsp od butter

1 tbsp of all-purpose flour

1 tbsp of Dijon mustard

½ cup of sweet cream

1 tsp of salt

½ tsp of red pepper flakes

Preparation:

Pour vegetable broth into a deep pot and bring it to a boil. Now, add kale and spinach and sprinkle with pepper for some extra flavor. Add more water if the vegetables are not covered with broth. Cover with a lid and reduce temperature to low. Cook for about 15 minutes, or until soften. Remove from the heat and set aside to cool.

Combine cream ingredients in a mixing bowl. Stir well to combine.

Transfer veggies to a serving plate or bowl, and spoon in the cream. Give it a final stir and sprinkle with some extra red pepper flakes.

Serve immediately.

Nutrition information per serving: Kcal: 213, Protein: 5.2g, Carbs: 15.5g, Fats: 14.6g

10.   Apple Cinnamon Oatmeal Pancake

Ingredients:

½ cup of plain flour, gluten-free

1 large egg

1 cup of coconut milk

½ Alfriston apple, grated

¼ cup of almonds, ground

1 tsp of vanilla extract

Cooking oil

Yogurt for topping

Preparation:

Combine all ingredients in a large bowl. Spread some cooking oil over a small, non-stick frying pan.

Pour about ½ cup of pancake mixture and cook for about three minutes on each side.

Top with one tablespoon of yogurt.

Nutrition information per serving: Kcal:298, Protein:31.4g, Carbs: 42.5g, Fats: 26.7g

11. Salmon with Worcestershire Sauce

Ingredients:

4 wild salmon steaks, chopped into bite-sized pieces

2 cups of vegetable broth

2 medium-sized carrots, sliced

1 medium-sized zucchini, peeled and sliced

1 medium-sized bell pepper, chopped

For dressing:

2 tbsp of Worcestershire sauce

1 tsp of apple cider vinegar

1 tbsp of lemon juice

1 tsp of salt

½ tsp of black pepper, ground

1 tbsp of fresh basil, finely chopped

Preparation:

Combine all dressing ingredients in a mixing bowl. Set aside for 15 minutes to allow all flavors to mingle.

Pour 2 cups of vegetable broth into a deep pot. Add salmon chops and vegetables. Season with salt and pepper to taste. Add water if the vegetables are not covered with broth. Cover with a lid and cook for 20 minutes on medium temperature. Remove from the heat and let it cool for a while.

Drain salmon and veggies and transfer to the serving plate. Drizzle with dressing and serve.

Enjoy!

Nutrition information per serving: Kcal: 162, Protein: 18.2g, Carbs: 12.8g, Fats: 5.4g

12.   Blueberry Peach Smoothie

Ingredients:

¼ cup of blueberries

1 large peach, pit removed and chopped

1 tbsp of chia seeds

1 cup of almond milk

1 tsp of saliva

Preparation:

Combine all ingredients in a blender. Mix until smooth and transfer to a serving glasses. Add some more chia seeds for some extra flavor and nutrients.

Serve!

Nutrition information per serving: Kcal: 335, Protein: 28.5g, Carbs: 37.3g, Fats: 10.1g

13.   Shrimp with Avocado & Eggs

Ingredients:

3 cups of shrimps, peeled and deveined

1 medium-sized avocado, ripe

1 ½ cup of brown rice, pre-cooked

2 free range eggs

1 tbsp of honey

2 tsp of olive oil

¼ tsp of red pepper, ground

1 tbsp of red wine vinegar

2 tbsp of sesame seeds

1 cup of red beans, pre-cooked

Preparation:

Heat up the olive oil in a large saucepan over a medium temperature. Add honey and stir well until it melts. Now add the shrimps and fry well for few minutes on each side. Season with pepper and remove from the saucepan. Use the same saucepan to fry eggs for about 2 minutes. Transfer to a plate and cut into strips.

In a small bowl, combine the rice with red wine vinegar and red beans. Top with egg strips, shrimps and avocado slices.

Nutrition information per serving: Kcal: 246, Protein: 26.5g, Carbs: 6.2g, Fats: 14.7g

14.　　Quick Summer Cold Soup

Ingredients:

2 medium-sized tomato, chopped

1 large cucumber, peeled and sliced

1 cup of arugula, chopped

1 tbsp of fresh basil, finely chopped

1 tbsp of fresh coriander, finely chopped

1 cup of buttermilk

1 tbsp of sour cream

½ tsp of black pepper, ground

1 tsp of salt

Preparation:

Combine buttermilk, sour cream,salt, pepper, basil, and coriander in large mixing bowl. Stir all well to combine and set aside.

Now, combine tomato, cucumber, and arugula in a food processor. Blend until you get a creamy mixture. Transfer the mixture to the buttermilk bowl and stir all well once again.

Refrigerate for 30 minutes before using.

Nutrition information per serving: Kcal: 155, Protein: 8.4g, Carbs: 16.7g, Fats: 8.2g

15.   Avocado Oil Baked Potato

Ingredients:

8 large potatoes, peeled and thickly sliced

3 free-range eggs, hard-boiled

1 cup of cottage cheese, crumbled

2 tbsp of avocado oil

1 tbsp of mustard

1 tsp of salt

½ tsp of red pepper, ground

Preparation:

Peel potatoes and cut into thick slices. Cook in boiling water for about 20-30 minutes, until tender. Remove from heat and allow it to cool for a while.

Meanwhile, boil the eggs for 10 minutes. You want hard-boiled eggs for this salad. Peel and cut eggs into slices.

Mix hard-boiled eggs and potatoes in a bowl. Add cottage cheese, avocado oil, mustard, salt and pepper. Stir well with a fork. Cover and chill for about an hour.

You can add ½ tbsp of dried parsley, but this is optional.

Nutrition information per serving: Kcal: 351, Protein: 4.7g, Carbs: 37.2g, Fats: 25.8g

16.   Celery with Dill Sauce

Ingredients:

7 oz of celery, cut into lengthwise strips

1 small cucumber, cut into lengthwise strips

1 small zucchini, cut into lengthwise strips

1 medium-sized bulb of fennel, cut into lengthwise strips

1 tbsp of lemon juice

½ tsp of salt

¼ tsp of black pepper, ground

For the sauce:

1 cup of Greek yogurt

3 tbsp of vegetable oil

2 tbsp of lemon juice

½ tsp of salt

¼ tsp of black pepper, ground

1 tsp of dill, finely chopped

Preparation:

Combine all sauce ingredients in a mixing bowl. Stir well and set aside.

Now, combine all vegetables on the serving plate. Serve sauce from the side, or simply spoon over the veggies.

Season with salt and pepper to taste.

Nutritional information per serving: Kcal: 105, Protein: 10.5g, Carbs: 14.6g, Fats: 6.3g

17.   Wild Green Soup

Ingredients:

4 oz of wild asparagus, chopped

2 oz of spinach, chopped

1 tbsp of fresh basil, chopped

2 garlic cloves, crushed

2 tbsp of vegetable oil

1 cup of milk

2 tbsp of fresh parsley, finely chopped

½ tsp of black pepper, ground

½ tsp of salt

Water

Preparation:

Combine spinach,milk, basil, and garlic in a blender. Blend until soften and set aside.

Now, place asparagus in a large pot and add one cup of water. Add the blended mixture, and oil. stir all well. Add more water if needed to make a creamy texture. Sprinkle with some salt and pepper. Cover with a lid, reduce the heat to low, and cook for 20 minutes. Remove from the heat and set aside to cool.

Stir in one tablespoon of sour cream for extra sour flavor. This is, however, optional.

Nutritional information per serving: Kcal: 105, Protein: 7.7g, Carbs: 13.8g, Fats: 4.5g

18.   Mediterranean Chicken

Ingredients:

2 lbs of chicken breasts, skinless and boneless, chopped into bite-sized pieces

4 garlic cloves, chopped

1 medium-sized onion, peeled and sliced

2 large tomatoes, chopped

2 tbsp of extra virgin olive oil

1 tbsp of fresh basil, finely chopped

½ tsp of black pepper, ground

½ tsp of salt

1 tsp of vegetable seasoning mix

2 cups of white rice

Preparation:

Preheat the oil in a large skillet over medium-high temperature. Add the onion and stir-fry until soften or translucent. Now, add the chicken chops and garlic.

Cook for about 10 minutes or until nicely golden brown color, stirring occasionally.

Meanwhile, place the tomatoes in a food processor.Add a pinch of salt and blend until smooth. Spoon in the mixture into the pan and reduce the temperature to low. Season with pepper. Cover with a lid and cook for 25 minutes. if the mixture too thick, add water occasionally. Remove from the heat and transfer to the serving plate.

Meanwhile, place the rice into the boiling water in a deep pot. Sprinkle with vegetable seasoning mix and cook for 15 minutes. Remove from the heat and drain.

Serve rice with meat and season with fresh basil.

Nutritional information per serving: Kcal: 553, Protein: 22.4g, Carbs: 41.2g, Fats: 22.1g

19.   Oatmeal Soup

Ingredients:

4 oz of oatmeal

1 large carrot, sliced

1 cup of celery, sliced

½ cup of parsley, finely chopped

1 small onion, sliced

3 tbsp of vegetable oil

1 tbsp of all-purpose flour

½ tsp of salt

½ tsp of black pepper, ground

½ cup of sour cream

Lukewarm water

Preparation:

Preheat the oil in a deep pot over a medium-high temperature. Add the onion and stir-fry until soften. Now add celery, carrot, and parsley and stir well to combine.

Stir in the flour and pour 2 cups of lukewarm water. Sprinkle with some salt and pepper and cover with a lid. Reduce temperature to low and cook for 15 minutes.

Add the oatmeal and check out the level of water. Add more if needed to desired density. Give it a good stir and cook for about 20 minutes more. Remove from the heat and add sour cream. Stir well and leave it for a while to cool.

Serve warm.

Nutritional information per serving: Kcal: 85, Protein: 3.2g, Carbs: 14.7g, Fats: 1.7g

20.   Spanish Omelet

Ingredients:

4 medium-sized potatoes, peeled and sliced

5 large eggs

1 small onion, diced

2 tbsp of olive oil

1 tbsp of fresh parsley, finely chopped

½ tsp of salt

½ tsp of black pepper, ground

Preparation:

Beat the eggs in a mixing bowl. Add a pinch of salt, pepper, and parsley and whisk all together. Set aside.

Preheat the oil in large frying pan over a medium-high temperature. Add the sliced potatoes and fry for about 5 minutes, until fork-tender or crisp. Add the onions and cook for 2 minutes more.

Stir in the eggs into the pan and spread equally over the potatoes. Cook for about 3-4 minutes more from both sides. Remove from the heat and slice the omelet into desired shapes or portions.

Serve with tomato slices or some other fresh vegetable.

Nutritional information per serving: Kcal: 157, Protein: 9.8g, Carbs: 28.7g, Fats: 3.6g

21.   Cooked Beets Salad

Ingredients:

4 medium-sized beets, peeled and chopped

1 cup of leek, chopped

2 tbsp of lemon juice

1 tsp of salt

½ tsp of black pepper, ground

2 tbsp of olive oil

1 cup of cottage cheese, crumbled

1 small carrot, shredded

1 tsp of parsley, finely chopped

Preparation:

Pour 3 cups of water in a large deep pot and bring it to a boil. Gently place the beets and cover with a lid. Reduce the temperature to low and cook until soften, or fork-tender. Remove from the heat and drain. Transfer the beets to the serving bowl.

Now, combine lemon juice, salt, pepper, and oil in a small mixing bowl. Stir well to combine. Set aside.

Add leeks and shredded carrot to the beets and stir well. Spoon in the dressing mixture and give it a final stir. Set aside for about 30 minutes to allow flavors to meld.

Just before serving, add cheese and fresh parsley.

Nutritional information per serving: Kcal: 161, Protein: 6.2g, Carbs: 13.4g, Fats: 6.8g

22.   No-Bake Protein Balls with Oats

Ingredients:

1 ½ cup of rolled oats

½ cup of peanut butter

¼ cup of almonds, minced

3 tbsp of honey

1 tbsp of chia seeds,

1 tbsp of vanilla extract, organic

3 cups of milk

Preparation:

Place one cup of rolled oats in a bowl. Add other dry ingredients and stir to combine.

Now add in peanut butter and honey. Mix well and gently pour in the milk and vanilla extract.

Shape the balls using your hands, top with the remaining oats and place in the refrigerator for about 30 minutes.

Nutritional information per serving: Kcal: 261, Protein: 21.2g, Carbs: 34.5g, Fats: 6.3g

23.   Brussel Sprouts with Kefir Dressing

Ingredients:

1 lb of Brussel sprouts, halved

5 garlic cloves, finely chopped

2 tbsp of olive oil

½ tsp of salt

¼ tsp of black pepper, ground

1 tbsp of butter

For dressing:

½ cup of kefir

1 tbsp of lemon juice

½ cup of arugula, finely chopped

½ tsp of salt

1 tbsp of olive oil

Preparation:

Preheat the oven to 400°F.

Place the Brussel sprouts in a pot of boiling water. Reduce the heat to low and cook for about 10 minutes, or until soften. Remove from the heat, drain, and set aside.

Melt butter in frying pan over a medium-high temperature. Add garlic and stir-fry until translucent. Add Brussel sprouts and sprinkle with some salt and pepper. Cook for 3 minutes and remove from the heat. Set aside to cool and transfer to the serving bowl.

Meanwhile, combine dressing ingredients in a medium-sized mixing bowl. Stir well to allow flavors to meld.

Drizzle the dressing over the Brussel sprouts and serve!

Nutritional information per serving: Kcal: 167, Protein: 6.3g, Carbs: 10.5g, Fats: 14.8g

24.   Shrimps Spaghetti with Veggies

Ingredients:

8 oz of shrimps, peeled and deveined

½ cup of celery, chopped

2 medium-sized carrots, sliced

2 garlic cloves, finely chopped

½ cup of leeks, finely chopped

1 tbsp of olive oil

1 lb of spaghetti (or fresh tagliatelle pasta)

1 tsp of parsley, finely chopped

1 tsp of salt

½ tsp of black pepper, ground

3 tbsp of Parmesan cheese, shredded

Preparation:

Use the package instructions to cook spaghetti. When finished, drain, and set aside.

Preheat the oil in a large frying skillet over a medium-high temperature. Add garlic, celery, and leeks. Cook for about

3 minutes and add shrimps. Reduce the heat and sprinkle with salt and pepper to taste. Cook for 5 minutes more stirring constantly. Add 2 cups of and cover with a lid. Cook for 15 minutes or until water evaporates. Remove from the heat and transfer to the spaghetti bowl. Stir in parsley and sprinkle with extra salt and pepper if needed.

Top with shredded parmesan cheese and serve.

Nutritional information per serving: Kcal: 220, Protein: 8.3g, Carbs: 44.4g, Fats: 9.8g

25.   Turmeric Pineapple Smoothie

Ingredients:

1 cup of pineapple, chopped

¼ cup of mango, chopped

¼ cup of Goji berries

½ cup of Greek yogurt

1 tsp of turmeric, ground

1 tsp of cinnamon, ground

1 tsp of coconut flour

½ tbsp of honey

Preparation:

Combine all ingredients in a blender. Blend for about 1 minute until you get a nice, creamy smoothie. Transfer the mixture to a large serving glasses and refrigerate for about 1 hour before serving.

Just before the serving, you can sprinkle the smoothie with some orange or lemon zest for some extra flavor.

Enjoy!

Nutritional information per serving: Kcal: 220, Protein: 5.6g, Carbs: 32.4g, Fats: 1.2g

26.   Crock Pot Turkey

Ingredients:

2 lbs of turkey breast, boneless and skinless, chopped

4 oz of spinach, chopped

1 tbsp of chili powder

2 cups of vegetable broth

2 tbsp of lemon juice

1 tsp of salt

1 tsp of black pepper, ground

2 tbsp of olive oil

Preparation:

Preheat the oil in a large pot over a medium-high temperature.

Meanwhile, wash and clean the meat. Sprinkle salt and pepper evenly to coat the meat.

Place the meat chops into the crock pot and cook meat for about 10 minutes. Now, add spinach, chili, and vegetable broth. If needed, pour water to cover all ingredients.

Reduce the heat to low and cover with a lid. Cook for 2 hours. Remove from the heat and leave it to cool.

Just before serving, drizzle the portion with lemon juice.

Place in a crock pot with other ingredients and cover. Cook for about 2 hours.

Nutrition information per serving: Kcal: 270, Protein: 35.5g, Carbs: 32.8g, Fats: 24.2g

27.   Raw Cocoa and Chia Seed Balls

Ingredients:

1 cup of minced almonds

½ cup of peanut butter

½ cup of honey

2 tablespoons of minced chia seeds

¼ cup of raw cocoa powder

¼ cup of grated dark chocolate, 85% cocoa

¼ cup of skim milk

Preparation:

Combine the ingredients in a bowl and mix well to combine. Shape the balls using your hands and refrigerate for about 30 minutes.

Nutritional information per serving: Kcal: 269, Protein: 24.4g, Carbs: 38.2g, Fats:8.5g

28.   Warm Squid Salad

Ingredients:

2 lbs of squids, cleaned, cut into bite-sized pieces

2 tbsp of lemon juice

1 cup of spring onions, chopped

2 medium-sized bell peppers, chopped

3 tbsp of olive oil

1 tsp of salt

½ tsp of black pepper, ground

Preparation:

Place squids into a large pot. Add enough water to cover. Cook on a medium temperature for about 15 minutes. Remove from the heat and drain. Transfer the squids to a large bowl.

Add spring onions, peppers, olive oil, salt, and pepper and give it a good stir. Set aside and cover for 2 hours to allow flavors to mingle.

Serve.

Nutrition information per serving: Kcal: 302, Protein: 35.2g, Carbs: 46.5g, Fats: 20.3g

29. Baked Eggs and Prosciutto in Portobello Mushrooms

Ingredients:

6 mushroom Portobello caps, cleaned, de-stemmed, scraped gills

6 strips of Prosciutto

6 large eggs

1 tsp of fresh parsley

3 tbsp of olive oil

½ tsp of salt

1 tsp of black pepper, ground

Preparation:

Your mushroom caps should be cleaned and cut into small bowl-like shapes. Take the caps and apply some olive oil on the outside to cook them easily and so that they will not stick to the baking sheet.

Line a baking tray with some baking paper before putting the mushroom caps on them. Take a slice of prosciutto and stuff it inside the mushroom cap. Make sure the slices fits neatly inside it.

Once you have stuffed all your mushroom caps with prosciutto, set them aside. Crack an egg into a small bowl and carefully, slide the egg inside the prosciutto stuffed mushroom cap. This step may take some time since the egg yolk can make the mushroom overturn or spill out.

Once all the eggs are in the mushroom caps, season with some salt, parsley, and pepper. Be careful of the salt since prosciutto is a rather salty meat and adding extra salt might make increase the saltiness of the dish.

Once you have seasoned everything, slide the baking tray extremely carefully into the oven. Be gentle to avoid overturning any mushroom caps. Once they're inside, let them cook for 30 minutes or until you feel the mushroom cap and egg are cooked to your liking.

Let them cool a bit before you take them out of the oven.

Serve:

Serve hot or cold with some sour cream and dill as garnishes.

Nutrition information per serving: Kcal: 134, Protein: 14.2g, Carbs: 0.7g, Fats: 7.8g

30.   Citrus Salmon

Ingredients:

1 lb of wild salmon filet, skinless and chopped into bite-sized pieces

3 tbsp of lemon juice

1 tbsp of olive oil

2 tbsp of all-purpose flour

2 oz of butter

4 oz of asparagus, whole

1 tbsp of lime juice

1 tsp of lime zest

1 tsp of salt

1 tsp of black pepper, ground

Preparation:

Place meat chops into a large bowl. Add flour, salt, and pepper and coat well using your hands.

Combine butter and oil in a large frying skillet over a medium-high temperature. Heat until butter melts and add meat chops. Cook for 15 minutes, or until golden brown. Transfer the meat to another dish and reserve the pan.

Add lemon juice, lime juice, and asparagus to skillet and cook for 5 minutes, stirring occasionally.

Return the salmon chops to the pan, add salt and pepper, and stir all to combine. Cook for 5 minutes and remove from the heat. Transfer all to a serving plate.

Top with a pinch of lime zest and serve.

Nutrition information **per serving:** Kcal: 282, Protein: 42.1g, Carbs: 7.5g, Fats: 12.2g

31.   Wild Berries Pancakes with Rice Flour

Ingredients:

1 cup of mixed wild berries, fresh

½ cup of rice flour

½ cup of skim milk

½ cup of almond milk

3 tbsp of honey

1 tsp of organic vanilla extract, powdered

1 tsp of baking powder

1 whole egg

½ cup of low-fat cream

½ cup of agave syrup

1 tbsp of sunflower oil

Preparation:

Combine flour, baking powder, skim milk and almond milk in a bowl and mix well with a fork, until smooth mixture.

In another bowl, mix the cream with 3 tbsp of honey, vanilla extract, and egg. Beat well with a fork, or even better with an electric mixer. You want to get a foamy mixture.

Whisk in this mixture in a first bowl to make a thick batter.

Cover it and let it stand for about 15 minutes.

Heat a tablespoon of sunflower oil in a non-stick frying pan.

Use ¼ cup of pancake mixture to make one pancake. You can use some pancake molds, but this is optional.

Fry your pancakes for about 2-3 minutes on each side. This mixture should give you 6 pancakes.

Spread 1 tbsp of agave syrup over each pancake, top with wild berries and serve.

Nutrition information per serving: Kcal: 312, Protein: 38.1, Carbs: 42.4g, Fats: 25.5g

32.   Tagliatelle in Melon Sauce

Ingredients:

1 lb of Tagliatelle pasta, pre-cooked

1 small melon, peeled, seeds removed and chopped

2 oz of butter

1 cup of sweet cream

½ tsp of salt

½ tsp of black pepper, ground

1 tsp of vegetable seasoning mix

¼ cup of Parmesan, shredded

1 tbsp of fresh parsley, finely chopped

Preparation:

Use the package instructions to cook pasta. Drain well and transfer to a large bowl.

Meanwhile, combine melon chops and sweet cream in a blender. Blend until smooth creamy mixture. Set aside.

Melt butter in a large frying skillet over a medium heat. Add melon cream mixture, salt, pepper, and vegetable seasoning mix. Pour ½ cup of lukewarm water and stir constantly. Cook for 10 minutes and remove from the heat.

Pour the sauce over the pasta and top with shredded Parmesan and parsley.

Nutrition information per serving: Kcal: 293, Protein: 9.6g, Carbs: 63.7g, Fats: 15.8g

33.   Brussels Sprouts in Coconut Gravy

Ingredients:

1 lb of Brussels sprouts

2 cup of coconut milk

4 onions, chopped

1 tbsp of olive oil

½ tsp of salt

½ tsp of black pepper, ground

½ cup of cashew paste

1 tbsp of fresh coriander, finely chopped

Preparation:

Heat up some olive oil in a large frying skillet. Add the onions and stir-fry for several minutes. Now add the Brussels sprouts and cashew paste. Reduce the heat to medium and fry for about 5 minutes.

Add the coconut milk, season with some salt and pepper and cover. Cook for about 10 minutes over a medium-low temperature.

Remove from the heat and top with the fresh coriander.

Nutrition information per serving: Kcal: 123, Protein: 4.5g, Carbs: 10.6g, Fats: g

34.   Spicy Vegetable Minestrone

Ingredients:

4 oz of green beans, halved

2 medium-sized carrots, sliced

1 cup of celery, chopped

1 cup of white beans

1 large zucchini, peeled and sliced

1 medium-sized onion, sliced

3 tbsp of vegetable oil

3 garlic cloves, chopped

1 tsp of fresh basil, chopped

1 tsp of chili, ground

1 tbsp of cayenne pepper, ground

1 tsp of fresh rosemary, crushed

1 cup of tomato sauce

1 tbsp of fresh parsley, finely chopped

1 tsp of vegetable seasoning mix

Preparation:

Preheat the oil in a deep pot over a medium-high temperature. Add garlic and onion and stir-fry for 2 minutes. Now add carrot, green beans, white beans, zucchinis, and celery. Sprinkle with salt and pepper and pour water enough to cover all ingredients. Cover with a lid and reduce the temperature to low. Cook for about 15 minutes and add tomato sauce and all remaining spices.

Cook for 1 hour and remove from the heat. Open the lid and let it cool for a while.

Just before serving, sprinkle with some fresh rosemary for extra taste.

Nutrition information per serving: Kcal: 120, Protein: g, Carbs: 63.7g, Fats: 15.8g

35.   Apple Cinnamon Oats

Ingredients:

½ cup gluten-free oats

1cup of water

1 Alkmene apple, peeled and grated

1 apple, sliced

2 tbsp of almond yogurt

1 tsp of cinnamon, ground

Preparation:

Boil the water and add oats. Briefly, cook (for several minutes) and reduce the heat.

Add one grated Alkmene apple and one teaspoon of cinnamon. Simmer for another ten minutes. Remove from the heat.

Top with almond yogurt and sliced apple. Serve warm.

Nutrition information per serving: Kcal: 120, Protein: 3.5g, Carbs: 25.8g, Fats: 1.3g

JUICES

1.   Ginger Carrot Juice

Ingredients:

1 medium-sized carrot

1 medium-sized apple, cored

1 large cucumber

1 large beet, trimmed

1 small ginger knob, 1 inch

Preparation:

Wash the carrot and cucumber and cut into thick slices. Set aside.

Wash the apple and remove the core. Cut into bite-sized pieces and set aside.

Wash the beet and trim off the green parts. Cut into small pieces and set aside.

Peel the ginger root knob and set aside.

Now, combine carrot, apple, cucumber, beet, and ginger in a juicer and process until juiced.

Transfer to serving glasses and add some ice cubes and serve immediately.

Enjoy!

Nutrition information per serving: Kcal: 166, Protein: 4.7g, Carbs: 48.4g, Fats: 0.9g

2.   Basil Honey Juice

Ingredients:

1 large artichoke heart

1 cup of avocado, cubed

1 large cucumber

1 cup of fresh basil

1 cup of green cabbage

1 tbsp of liquid honey

Preparation:

Using a sharp knife, trim off the outer leaves of the artichoke. Wash it and cut into small pieces. Set aside.

Peel the avocado and cut in half. Remove the pit and cut into cubes. Reserve the rest of the avocado for some other juice. Set aside.

Wash the cucumber and cut into thick slices. Set aside.

Wash the basil and cabbage thoroughly and torn with hands. Set aside.

Now, process artichoke, avocado, cucumber, basil, and cabbage in a juicer. Transfer to serving glasses and stir in the liquid honey.

Refrigerate for 30 minutes before serving.

Nutrition information per serving: Kcal: 357, Protein: 12.1g, Carbs: 63.6g, Fats: 22.8g

3.   Spinach Pomegranate Juice

Ingredients:

1 bunch of fresh spinach

1 cup of pomegranate seeds

1 cup of fresh kale

1 large lemon, peeled

1 cup of watercress

1 cup of Swiss chard

Preparation:

Combine spinach, kale, watercress, and Swiss chard in a colander. Wash thoroughly under cold running water. Drain and torn with hands. Set aside.

Cut the top of the pomegranate fruit using a sharp knife. Slice down to each of the white membranes inside of the fruit. Pop the seeds into a bowl and set aside.

Peel the lemon and cut lengthwise in half. Set aside.

Now, process spinach, kale, watercress, Swiss chard, pomegranate seeds, and lemon in a juicer.

Transfer to serving glasses and add few ice cubes before serving.

Enjoy!

Nutrition information per serving: Kcal: 357, Protein: 12.1g, Carbs: 63.6g, Fats: 22.8g

4.   Asparagus Pepper Juice

Ingredients:

2 cups of fresh asparagus, trimmed

1 large fennel bulb, trimmed

1 large green bell pepper, seeded

1 large yellow bell pepper, seeded

1 ginger root slice, 1-inch

2 oz of water

Preparation:

Wash the asparagus and trim off the woody ends. Cut into 1-inch pieces and set aside.

Wash the fennel bulb and trim off the wilted outer layers. Cut into small chunks and set aside.

Wash the bell peppers and cut in half. Remove the seeds and cut into small slices. Set aside.

Peel the ginger root slice and set aside.

Now, combine asparagus, fennel, green and yellow bell pepper, and ginger root in a juicer and process until juiced.

Transfer to serving glasses and stir in the water. Refrigerate for 10 minutes before serving and enjoy!

Nutrition information per serving: Kcal: 143, Protein: 12.1g, Carbs: 47.2g, Fats: 1.5g

5.   Honeydew Parsnip Juice

Ingredients:

1 large wedge of honeydew melon

1 cup of Brussels sprouts, trimmed

1 cup of parsnip, trimmed

1 cup of fresh broccoli

1 medium-sized apple, cored

2 oz of water

Preparation:

Cut the honeydew melon lengthwise in half. Scoop out the seeds using a spoon. Cut one large wedge and peel it. Cut into small chunks and place in a bowl. Wrap the rest of the melon in a plastic foil and refrigerate.

Wash the Brussels sprouts and trim off the outer leaves. Cut in half and set aside.

Wash the parsnips and cut into thick slices. Fill into the measuring cup and reserve the rest for some other juice. Set aside.

Wash the broccoli and chop into small pieces. Set aside.

Wash the apple and remove the core. Cut into bite-sized pieces and set aside.

Now, process honeydew melon, Brussels sprouts, parsnips, broccoli, and apple in a juicer.

Transfer to serving glasses and stir in the water. Add some ice and serve!

Nutrition information per serving: Kcal: 251, Protein: 8.7g, Carbs: 75.1g, Fats: 1.5g

6. Broccoli Mustard Greens Juice

Ingredients:

2 cups of fresh broccoli

1 cup of mustard greens

1 large grapefruit

1 cup of Romaine lettuce

1 medium-sized zucchini

2 oz of water

Preparation:

Wash the broccoli and chop into small pieces. Set aside.

Combine mustard greens and Romaine lettuce in a colander. Wash under cold running water and torn with hands. Set aside.

Peel the grapefruit and divide into wedges. Set aside.

Peel the zucchini and cut in half. Scrape out the seeds and cut into small chunks. Set aside.

Now, process broccoli, mustard greens, grapefruit, lettuce, and zucchini in a juicer. Transfer to serving glasses and add some ice.

Serve immediately.

Nutrition information per serving: Kcal: 166, Protein: 11.6g, Carbs: 48.6g, Fats: 2.1g

7.   Orange Cantaloupe Juice

Ingredients:

2 large oranges, peeled

1 cup of cantaloupe, cubed

2 medium-sized radishes, trimmed

1 ginger root knob, 1-inch

1 tbsp of liquid honey

2 oz of water

Preparation:

Peel the oranges and divide into wedges. Set aside.

Cut the cantaloupe in half. Scoop out the seeds and flesh. You will need about one large wedge for one cup. Cut and peel it. Chop into chunks and set aside. Reserve the rest of the cantaloupe in a refrigerator.

Wash the radishes and trim off the green parts. Cut into small pieces and set aside.

Peel the ginger root knob and set aside.

Now, process oranges, cantaloupe, radishes, and ginger in a juicer. Transfer to serving glasses and stir in the honey and water.

Add few ice cubes or refrigerate for 10 minutes before serving.

Nutrition information per serving: Kcal: 250, Protein: 4.9g, Carbs: 74.3g, Fats: 0.8g

8.   Italian Tomato Juice

Ingredients:

2 large tomatoes

1 cup of fresh basil

1 cup of fresh celery, chopped

½ tsp of Himalayan salt

½ tsp of dried oregano, ground

Preparation:

Wash the tomatoes and place them in a bowl. Cut into quarters and reserve the juice while cutting. Set aside.

Combine basil and celery in a colander and wash under cold running water. Torn with hands and set aside.

Now, combine tomatoes, basil, and celery in a juicer and process until juiced.

Transfer to serving glasses and stir in the reserved tomato juice, salt. Sprinkle with some oregano for some extra taste.

Refrigerate for 10 minutes before serving.

Nutrition information per serving: Kcal: 64, Protein: 4.6g, Carbs: 17.8g, Fats: 1.1g

9. Coconut Papaya Juice

Ingredients:

1 large papaya, seeded and peeled

2 large carrots

1 large lime, peeled

2 oz of coconut water

Preparation:

Peel the papaya and cut lengthwise in half. Scoop out the black seeds and flesh using a spoon. Cut into small chunks. Set aside.

Wash the carrots and cut into thick slices. Set aside.

Peel the lime and cut lengthwise in half. Set aside.

Now, combine papaya, carrots, and lime in a juicer and process until juiced.

Transfer to serving glasses and stir in the coconut water. Add few ice cubes or refrigerate before serving.

Enjoy!

Nutrition information per serving: Kcal: 347, Protein: 5.2g, Carbs: 119g, Fats: 2.4g

10.   Yellow Juice

Ingredients:

1 large zucchini chunks

1 large lemon, peeled

1 cup of pumpkin

1 medium-sized yellow apple, cored

1 medium-sized banana

2 oz of water

Preparation:

Peel the zucchini and cut in half. Scrape out the seeds with a spoon. Cut into chunks and set aside.

Peel the lemon and cut lengthwise in half. Set aside.

Peel the pumpkin and cut in half. Scoop out the seeds using a spoon. Cut one large wedge and peel it. Cut into small chunks and set aside. Reserve the rest for later.

Wash the apple and remove the core. Cut into bite-sized pieces and set aside.

Peel the banana and cut into small chunks. Set aside.

Now, process zucchini, lemon, pumpkin, apple, and banana in a juicer. Transfer to serving glasses and stir in the water.

Add some ice and serve immediately.

Nutrition information per serving: Kcal: 254, Protein: 7.5g, Carbs: 72.9g, Fats: 1.9g

11.   Chia Juice

Ingredients:

1 large cucumber

1 large lemon, peeled

1 large lime, peeled

1 large orange, peeled

1 tbsp of chia seeds

2 oz of water

Preparation:

Wash the cucumber and cut into thick slices. Set aside.

Peel the lemon and lime and cut lengthwise in half. Set aside.

Peel the orange and divide into wedges. Set aside.

Now, combine cucumber, lemon, lime, and orange in a juicer and process until juiced.

Transfer to serving glasses and stir in some chia seeds for some extra nutrients.

Add few ice cubes and refrigerate for 20 minutes before serving.

Stir in the water after refrigerating and enjoy!

Nutrition information per serving: Kcal: 186, Protein: 6.2g, Carbs: 41.4g, Fats: 5g

12.   Swiss Chard Celery Juice

Ingredients:

1 cup of Swiss chards

1 cup of celery

1 medium-sized apple, cored

1 cup of collard greens

2 tbsp of fresh parsley

4-5 fresh spinach leaves

2 oz of water

Preparation:

Combine Swiss chards, collard greens, celery, and spinach in a colander. Wash thoroughly under cold running water and drain. Torn with hands and set aside.

Wash the apple and remove the core. Cut into bite-sized pieces and set aside.

Now, combine Swiss chards, celery, apple, collard greens, and spinach in a juicer and process until juiced.

Transfer to serving glasses and stir in the water. Add some ice and garnish with fresh parsley.

Enjoy!

Nutrition information per serving: Kcal: 106, Protein: 4.8g, Carbs: 31.3g, Fats: 1.1g

13.   Watermelon Watercress Juice

Ingredients:

1 cup of watermelon, seeded

1 cup of watercress

2 large leeks

1 large lemon, peeled

1 cup of beet greens

2 oz of water

Preparation:

Cut the watermelon lengthwise. For two cups, you will need about two large wedges. Peel and cut into chunks. Remove the seeds and set aside. Reserve the rest of the melon for some other juices.

Wash the watercress and beet greens thoroughly under cold running water and torn with hands. Set aside.

Wash the leeks and cut into 1-inch pieces. Set aside.

Peel the lemon and cut lengthwise in half. Set aside.

Now, combine watermelon, watercress, leeks, lemon, and beet greens in a juicer and process until juiced.

Transfer to serving glasses and stir in the water. Add some ice cubes and serve immediately.

Nutrition information per serving: Kcal: 156, Protein: 5.9g, Carbs: 44.2g, Fats: 1.1g

14.　Blueberry Butternut Squash Juice

Ingredients:

1 cup of blueberries

1 large orange, peeled

1 cup of butternut squash

1 medium-sized apple, cored

1 large kiwi, peeled

2 tbsp of fresh parsley

Preparation:

Place the blueberries in a colander and wash under cold running water. Drain and set aside.

Peel the orange and divide into wedges. Set aside.

Peel the butternut squash and remove the seeds using a spoon. Cut into small cubes and reserve the rest of the squash for some other recipe. Wrap in a plastic foil and refrigerate.

Wash the apple and remove the core. Cut into bite-sized pieces and set aside.

Peel the kiwi and cut lengthwise in half. Set aside.

Now, process blueberries, orange, butternut squash, apple, and kiwi in a juicer.

Transfer to serving glasses and garnish with parsley.

Refrigerate for 10 minutes before serving.

Nutrition information per serving: Kcal: 304, Protein: 5.9g, Carbs: 92.4g, Fats: 1.6g

15.   Strawberry Beet Juice

Ingredients:

1 cup of fresh strawberries

1 cup of beets, trimmed

1 large red apple, cored

1 large lime, peeled

1 ginger root knob, 1-inch

1 tbsp of liquid honey

2 oz of water

Preparation:

Place the strawberries in a colander and wash under cold running water. Drain and cut in half. Set aside.

Wash the beets and trim off the green parts. Cut into small pieces and fill the measuring cup. Reserve the beet greens for some other juice. Set aside.

Wash the apple and remove the core. Cut into bite-sized pieces. Set aside.

Peel the lime and cut lengthwise in half. Set aside.

Peel the ginger root knob and set aside.

Now, combine strawberries, beets, apple, and ginger in a juicer and process until juiced.

Transfer to serving glasses and stir in honey and water. Add some ice and serve immediately.

Nutrition information per serving: Kcal: 277, Protein: 4.2g, Carbs: 82.4g, Fats: 1.3g

16.   Sweet Potato Spinach Juice

Ingredients:

1 cup of sweet potatoes, cubed

1 bunch of fresh spinach

1 large cucumber

1 ginger root knob, 1-inch

Preparation:

Peel the sweet potatoes and cut into small cubes. Fill the measuring cup and reserve the rest for some other juice. Set aside.

Wash the spinach thoroughly under cold running water and torn with hands. Set aside.

Wash the cucumber and cut into thick slices. Set aside.

Peel the ginger root knob and set aside.

Now, combine sweet potatoes, spinach, cucumber and ginger root in a juicer and process until juiced.

Transfer to serving glasses stir in the water. Refrigerate for 15 minutes before serving.

Nutrition information per serving: Kcal: 190, Protein: 13.8g, Carbs: 51.1g, Fats: 1.7g

17.   Brussels Sprout Juice

Ingredients:

1 cup of Brussels sprouts, trimmed

1 cup of fresh broccoli

1 large artichoke head

1 large lemon, peeled

1 large cucumber

3 tbsp of fresh parsley

Preparation:

Wash the Brussels sprouts and trim off the outer layers. Cut in half and set aside.

Wash the broccoli and chop into small pieces. set aside.

Using a sharp knife, trim off the outer layers of the artichoke. Wash it and cut into bite-sized pieces. Set aside.

Peel the lemon and cut lengthwise in half. Set aside.

Wash the cucumber and cut into thick slices. Set aside.

Now, process Brussels sprouts, broccoli, artichoke, lemon, and cucumber in a juicer.

Transfer to serving glasses and garnish with fresh parsley. Refrigerate for 10 minutes before serving.

Enjoy!

Nutrition information per serving: Kcal: 140, Protein: 13.8g, Carbs: 48.1g, Fats: 1.4g

18.   Green Bean Juice

Ingredients:

1 cup of green beans

1 cup of asparagus, trimmed

1 cup of fresh celery

1 large cucumber

1 cup of Romaine lettuce

1 large apple, cored

1 oz of water

Preparation:

Wash the green beans and cut into 1-inch pieces. Set aside.

Wash the asparagus and trim off the woody ends. Cut into small pieces and set aside.

Wash the celery and cut into bite-sized pieces. Set aside.

Wash the cucumber and cut into thick slices. Set aside.

Wash the lettuce thoroughly under cold running water. Drain and torn with hands. Set aside.

Wash the apple and remove the core. Cut into bite-sized pieces and set aside.

Now, process green beans, asparagus, celery, cucumber, lettuce and apple in a juicer. Transfer to serving glasses and stir in some water.

Add some ice and serve.

Nutrition information per serving: Kcal: 185, Protein: 8.1g, Carbs: 52.5g, Fats: 1.3g

19.　Pumpkin Rosemary Juice

Ingredients:

1 cup of pumpkin, cubed

1 large yellow bell pepper, seeded

1 large orange, peeled

1 large lime, peeled

1 small rosemary sprig

Preparation:

Peel the pumpkin and cut in half. Scoop out the seeds using a spoon. Cut one large wedge and peel it. Cut into small chunks and fill the measuring cup. Reserve the rest for some other juice.

Wash the bell pepper and cut in half. Remove the seeds and cut into small slices. Set aside.

Peel the orange and divide into wedges. Set aside.

Peel the lime and cut lengthwise in half. Set aside.

Now, combine pumpkin, bell pepper, orange, and lime in a juicer and process until juiced. Transfer to serving glasses and sprinkle with some rosemary to taste.

Refrigerate for 15 minutes before serving.

Nutrition information per serving: Kcal: 149, Protein: 4.9g, Carbs: 44.6g, Fats: 0.7g

20.   Mint Lime Juice

Ingredients:

1 cup of fresh mint

1 large lime, peeled

2 large honeydew melon wedges

1 large yellow apple, cored

2 oz of coconut water

Preparation:

Wash the mint thoroughly under cold running water. Drain and torn with hands. Set aside.

Peel the lime and cut lengthwise in half. Set aside.

Cut the honeydew melon lengthwise in half. Scoop out the seeds using a spoon. Cut two large wedges and peel them. Cut into small chunks and place in a bowl. Wrap the rest of the melon in a plastic foil and refrigerate.

Wash the apple and remove the core. Cut into bite-sized pieces and set aside.

Now, combine mint, lime, honeydew melon, and apple in a juicer. Transfer to serving glasses and stir in the coconut water.

Add some ice and serve immediately.

Nutrition information per serving: Kcal: 228, Protein: 3.4g, Carbs: 65.7g, Fats: 1g

21.   Grapefruit Raspberry Juice

Ingredients:

1 large grapefruit, peeled

1 cup of raspberries

1 large carrot

1 medium-sized apple, cored

1 small ginger root slice, 1-inch

1 oz of water

Preparation:

Peel the grapefruit and divide into wedges. Set aside.

Place the raspberries in a colander and wash under cold running water. Drain and set aside.

Wash the carrot and cut into thick slices. Set aside.

Wash the apple and remove the core. Cut into bite-sized pieces. Set aside.

Peel the ginger root and set aside.

Now, process grapefruit, raspberries, carrot, apple, and ginger in a juicer.

Transfer to serving glasses and stir in the water. Add few ice cubes or refrigerate before serving.

Enjoy!

Nutrition information per serving: Kcal: 239, Protein: 4.9g, Carbs: 76.2g, Fats: 1.7g

22.   Pineapple Cabbage Juice

Ingredients:

1 cup of pineapple chunks

1 cup of purple cabbage, chopped

1 large beet, trimmed

1 large carrot

A handful of fresh spinach

1 tbsp of liquid honey

Preparation:

Cut the top of a pineapple and peel it using a sharp knife. Cut into small chunks and fill the measuring cup. Reserve the rest of the pineapple in a refrigerator.

Wash the purple cabbage and spinach thoroughly torn with hands. Set aside.

Wash the beet and trim off the green parts. Cut into small pieces and set aside.

Wash the carrot and cut into thick slices. Set aside.

Now, process pineapple, cabbage, beet, carrot, and spinach in a juicer.

Transfer to serving glasses and stir in the liquid honey. Add few ice cubes and serve immediately.

Enjoy!

Nutrition information per serving: Kcal: 205, Protein: 5g, Carbs: 62.1g, Fats: 0.7g

23.   Fuji Juice

Ingredients:

2 medium-sized Fuji apples

1 large lemon, peeled

1 large cucumber

3 medium-sized celery stalks

A handful of spinach

2 oz of water

Preparation:

Wash the apples and remove the core. Cut into bite-sized pieces and set aside.

Peel the lemon and cut lengthwise in half. Set aside.

Wash the cucumber and cut into thick slices. Set aside.

Wash the celery stalks and cut into 1-inch pieces. Set aside.

Wash the spinach thoroughly and torn with hands. Set aside.

Now, process apples, lemon, cucumber, celery, and spinach in a juicer. Transfer to serving glasses and stir in the water.

Add some ice and serve.

Nutrition information per serving: Kcal: 224, Protein: 5.2g, Carbs: 65.4g, Fats: 1.5g

24.   Zucchini Pear Juice

Ingredients:

1 medium-sized zucchini

1 large pear, cored

1 cup of fresh broccoli, chopped

1 large fennel bulb

1 small ginger root slice

Preparation:

Peel the zucchini and cut in half. Scrape out the seeds with a spoon. Cut into chunks and set aside.

Wash the pear and remove the core. Cut into small pieces and set aside.

Wash the broccoli and cut into small pieces and set aside.

Trim off the outer leaves of the artichoke using a sharp knife. Cut into small pieces and set aside.

Peel the ginger root and set aside.

Now, process zucchini, pear, broccoli, fennel, and ginger in a juicer.

Transfer to serving glasses and add some ice before serving.

Nutrition information per serving: Kcal: 195, Protein: 8.7g, Carbs: 64.5g, Fats: 1.8g

25.   Parsley Juice

Ingredients:

1 cup of fresh parsley, torn

2 cups of Swiss chard

1 large cucumber

1 small yellow apple, cored

1 small orange, peeled

Preparation:

Combine parsley and Swiss chard in a colander and wash thoroughly under cold running water. Drain and torn with hands. Set aside.

Wash the cucumber and cut into thick slices. Set aside.

Wash the apple and remove the core. Cut into bite-sized pieces and set aside.

Peel the orange and divide into wedges. Set aside.

Now, combine parsley, Swiss chard, cucumber apple, and orange in a juicer and process until juiced. Transfer to serving glasses and add some ice before serving.

Enjoy!

Nutrition information per serving: Kcal: 161, Protein: 6.3g, Carbs: 46.3g, Fats: 1.2g

26.   Jalapeno Watermelon Juice

Ingredients:

2 cups of watermelon, seeded

1 cup of Romaine lettuce, chopped

1 large orange, peeled

1 cup of fresh basil, chopped

¼ tsp of jalapeno pepper, ground

Preparation:

Cut the watermelon lengthwise. For two cups, you will need about two large wedges. Peel and cut into chunks. Remove the seeds and set aside. Reserve the rest of the melon for some other juices.

Combine lettuce and basil in a colander and wash under cold running water. Drain and chop into small pieces. Set aside.

Peel the orange and divide into wedges. Set aside.

Now, process watermelon, lettuce, basil, and orange in a juicer.

Transfer to serving glasses and stir in the jalapeno pepper for some extra spicy flavor. Refrigerate for 15 minutes before serving.

Enjoy!

Nutrition information per serving: Kcal: 165, Protein: 4.9g, Carbs: 46.7g, Fats: 1g

27.   Arugula Juice

Ingredients:

1 cup of fresh arugula

1 cup of fresh mint

1 large carrot

1 large orange, peeled

1 large red bell pepper, seeded

Preparation:

Combine arugula and mint in a colander and wash thoroughly under cold running water. Drain and torn with hands. Set aside.

Wash the carrot and cut into thick slices. Set aside.

Peel the orange and divide into wedges. Set aside.

Wash the bell pepper and cut in half. Remove the seeds and chop into small slices. Set aside.

Now, combine arugula, mint, carrot, orange, and bell pepper in a juicer and process until juiced.

Transfer to serving glasses and stir in the water. You can add a pinch of Himalayan salt, but this is optional.

Add some ice and serve immediately.

Nutrition information per serving: Kcal: 153, Protein: 7.9g, Carbs: 47.3g, Fats: 1.3g

28.   Mixed Greens Juice

Ingredients:

1 cup of collard greens, chopped

1 cup of Swiss chard, chopped

1 cup of red leaf lettuce, chopped

1 cup of Romaine lettuce, chopped

1 large cucumber

1 large orange, peeled

1 large lemon, peeled

2 oz of water

Preparation:

Combine collard greens, Swiss chard, red leaf lettuce, and Romaine lettuce in a colander. Wash under cold running water and drain. Torn with hands and set aside.

Wash the cucumber and cut into thick slices. Set aside.

Peel the orange and divide into wedges. Set aside.

Peel the lemon and cut lengthwise in half. Set aside.

Now, process collard greens, Swiss chard, red leaf lettuce, Romaine lettuce, cucumber, orange, and lemon in a juicer.

Transfer to serving glasses and stir in the water.

Add some ice and serve immediately.

Nutrition information per serving: Kcal: 136, Protein: 7g, Carbs: 43.4g, Fats: 1.2g

29.   Broccoli Plum Juice

Ingredients:

5 large plums, pitted

1 cup of fresh broccoli

1 large cucumber

1 medium-sized apple, cored

Preparation:

Wash the plums and cut in half. Remove the pits and set aside.

Wash the broccoli and cut into small pieces. Set aside.

Wash the cucumber and cut into thick slices and set aside.

Wash the apple and remove the core. Cut into bite-sized pieces and set aside.

Now, combine plums, broccoli, cucumber, and apple in a juicer and process until juiced.

Transfer to serving glasses and add few ice cubes before serving.

Enjoy!

Nutrition information per serving: Kcal: 268, Protein: 7.6g, Carbs: 77.4g, Fats: 1.9g

30.   Sweet Apricot Juice

Ingredients:

1 cup of apricots, pitted and halved

1 large lemon, peeled

1 large carrot

1 medium-sized green apple, cored

1 tbsp of liquid honey

2 oz of water

Preparation:

Wash the apricots and cut in half. Remove the pits and fill the measuring cup. Reserve the rest for some other juice. Set aside.

Peel the lemon and cut lengthwise in half. Set aside.

Wash the carrot and cut into thick slices and set aside.

Wash the apple and remove the core. Cut into bite-sized pieces and set aside.

Now, combine apricots, lemon, carrot, and apple in a juicer and process until juiced.

Transfer to serving glasses and stir in the liquid honey and water.

Refrigerate for 15 minutes before serving.

Nutrition information per serving: Kcal: 243, Protein: 4.2g, Carbs: 69.3g, Fats: 1.3g

31. Mango Kale Juice

Ingredients:

1 cup of mango, chopped

1 cup of fresh kale

1 large artichoke head

1 large cucumber

1 ginger root knob, 1 inch

2 oz of water

Preparation:

Wash the mango and cut into small chunks. Fill the measuring cup and reserve the rest for some other juice. Set aside.

Wash the kale thoroughly and torn with hands. Set aside.

Wash the cucumber and cut into thick slices. Set aside.

Peel the ginger root knob and set aside.

Now, process mango, kale, cucumber, and ginger in a juicer.

Transfer to serving glasses and stir in the water. Add some ice and serve.

Enjoy!

Nutrition information per serving: Kcal: 197, Protein: 11.6g, Carbs: 59.6g, Fats: 1.8g

32. Green Cayenne Juice

Ingredients:

1 cup of fresh broccoli

1 large carrot

1 large leek

1 cup of kale, chopped

1 large lime, peeled

1 large lemon, peeled

1 large cucumber

¼ tsp of Cayenne pepper, ground

Preparation:

Wash the broccoli and cut into small pieces and set aside.

Wash the carrot and cucumber and cut into thick slices. Set aside.

Wash the kale and celery thoroughly under cold running water. Roughly chop it and set aside.

Peel the lemon and lime and cut lengthwise in half. Set aside.

Now, process broccoli, carrot, kale, leek, lemon, and lime in a juicer.

Transfer to serving glasses and stir in the Cayenne pepper for extra spicy flavor.

Refrigerate for 30 minutes before serving.

Nutrition information per serving: Kcal: 174, Protein: 10.2g, Carbs: 51.4g, Fats: 1.9g

33. Winter Squash Juice

Ingredients:

2 cups of butternut squash, seeded

2 large carrots

1 large Granny Smith Apple

1 small ginger root slice

Preparation:

Peel the butternut squash and remove the seeds using a spoon. Cut into small cubes and fill the measuring cup. Reserve the rest of the squash for some other juice. Wrap in a plastic foil and refrigerate.

Wash the carrots and cut into thick slices. Set aside.

Wash the apple and remove the core. Cut into bite-sized pieces and set aside.

Peel the ginger slice and set aside.

Now, process butternut squash, carrots, apple, and ginger in a juicer.

Transfer to serving glasses and refrigerate before serving.

Nutrition information per serving: Kcal: 246, Protein: 5.1g, Carbs: 75g, Fats: 1.1g

34.   Radish Beet Juice

Ingredients:

1 large orange, peeled

1 cup of beets, trimmed and chopped

1 large radish, chopped

1 cup of fresh kale, chopped

1 large cucumber

Preparation:

Peel the orange and divide into wedges. Set aside.

Wash the beets and trim off the green parts. Chop into bite-sized pieces and set aside.

Wash the radish and trim off the green parts. Cut into small pieces and set aside.

Wash the kale thoroughly under cold running water. Drain and torn with hands. Set aside.

Wash the cucumber and cut into thick slices. Set aside.

Now, combine orange, beets, radish, kale, and cucumber in a juicer and process until juiced.

Transfer to serving glasses and add some ice before serving.

Enjoy!

Nutrition information per serving: Kcal: 174, Protein: 8.8g, Carbs: 51.7g, Fats: 1.4g

35.   Fennel Greens Juice

Ingredients:

1 large fennel bulb

1 large yellow apple, cored

1 cup of fresh kale, chopped

1 cup of mustard greens

1 large bell pepper, seeded

Preparation:

Wash the fennel bulb and trim off the wilted outer layers. Cut into small chunks and set aside.

Wash the apple and remove the core. Cut into bite-sized pieces and set aside.

Combine kale and mustard greens in a colander. Wash under cold running water and torn with hands. Set aside.

Wash the bell pepper and cut in half. Remove the seeds and chop into small slices. Set aside.

Now, process fennel, apple, kale, mustard greens, and bell pepper in a juicer.

Transfer to serving glasses and refrigerate for 10 minutes before serving.

Nutrition information per serving: Kcal: 199, Protein: 9.4g, Carbs: 62.4g, Fats: 1.9g

36.   Summer Peach Juice

Ingredients:

2 large peaches, pitted and halved

1 cup of apricots, pitted and halved

1 cup of cantaloupe, chopped

3 oz of coconut water

Preparation:

Wash the peaches and cut in half. Remove the pits and cut into bite-sized pieces. Set aside.

Wash the apricots and cut in half. Remove the pits and fill the measuring cup. Reserve the rest for some other juice. Set aside.

Cut the cantaloupe in half. Scoop out the seeds and cut about two large wedges. Peel and chop into chunks. Fill the measuring cup and reserve the rest of the cantaloupe in a refrigerator for some other juice.

Now, process peaches, apricots, and cantaloupe in a juicer.

Transfer to serving glasses and stir in the coconut water. Add some ice and serve immediately.

Enjoy!

Nutrition information per serving: Kcal: 239, Protein: 6.8g, Carbs: 66.4g, Fats: 1.8g

37.   Brussels Sprout Asparagus Juice

Ingredients:

1 cup of asparagus, trimmed

1 cup of Brussels sprouts, trimmed

1 large tomato

1 cup of Swiss chard

1 large cucumber

Preparation:

Wash the asparagus and trim off the woody ends. Cut into 1-inch pieces and set aside.

Wash the Brussels sprouts and trim off the outer layers. Cut in half and set aside.

Wash the tomato and place in a bowl. Cut into quarters and reserve the juice while cutting. Set aside.

Wash the Swiss chard thoroughly under cold running water. Drain and set aside.

Wash the cucumber and cut into thick slices. Set aside.

Now, process asparagus, Brussels sprouts, tomato, Swiss chard, and cucumber in a juicer.

Transfer to serving glasses and add some ice before serving.

Nutrition information per serving: Kcal: 109, Protein: 10.1g, Carbs: 32.4g, Fats: 1.2g

38.   Beets & Grapes Juice

Ingredients:

3 large beets, trimmed

2 cups of green grapes

1 cup of cauliflower, chopped

1 large lemon, peeled

Preparation:

Wash the beets and trim off the green parts. Cut into bite-sized pieces and set aside.

Wash the green grapes under cold running water. Set aside.

Trim off the outer leaves of cauliflower. Wash it and cut into small pieces. Fill the measuring cup and reserve the rest for some other juice. Set aside.

Peel the lemon and cut lengthwise in half. Set aside.

Now, process beets, grapes, cauliflower, and lemon in a juicer.

Transfer to serving glasses and add some ice cubes before serving.

Enjoy!

Nutrition information per serving: Kcal: 226, Protein: 7.8g, Carbs: 65.8g, Fats: 1.5g

39.   Turnip Greens Juice

Ingredients:

1 cup of turnip greens, chopped

1 cup of kale, chopped

1 cup of Romaine lettuce, chopped

1 cup of cauliflower, chopped

1 large cucumber

Preparation:

Combine turnip greens, kale, and Romaine lettuce in a colander and wash under cold running water. Drain and roughly chop it. Set aside.

Trim off the outer leaves of cauliflower. Wash it and cut into small pieces. Fill the measuring cup and reserve the rest for some other juice. Set aside.

Wash the cucumber and cut into thick slices. Set aside.

Now, combine turnip greens, kale, Romaine lettuce, cauliflower, and cucumber in a juicer and process until juiced.

Transfer to serving glasses and add some ice before serving.

Enjoy!

Nutrition information per serving: Kcal: 96, Protein: 8.3g, Carbs: 27.6g, Fats: 1.6g

40.   Cranberry Apple Juice

Ingredients:

1 cup of cranberries

1 large red apple, cored

1 large lime, peeled

1 large orange, peeled

1 small ginger root knob, 1-inch

Preparation:

Place the cranberries in a colander and wash under cold running water. Drain and set aside.

Wash the apple and remove the core. Cut into bite-sized pieces and set aside.

Peel the lime and cut lengthwise in half. Set aside.

Peel the orange and divide into wedges. Set aside.

Peel the ginger knob and set aside.

Now, process cranberries, apple, lime, orange, and ginger in a juicer.

Transfer to serving glasses and refrigerate for 15 minutes before serving.

Enjoy!

Nutrition information per serving: Kcal: 240, Protein: 3.1g, Carbs: 75.1g, Fats: 0.9g

41.   Tomato Avocado Juice

Ingredients:

1 large tomato

1 cup of avocado, chopped

1 large cucumber

1 large lemon, peeled

1 cup of fresh basil, chopped

Preparation:

Wash the tomato and place in a bowl. Cut into quarters and reserve the juice while cutting. Set aside.

Peel the avocado and cut in half. Remove the pit and cut into chunks. Fill the measuring cup and reserve the rest for some other juice. Keep it in a refrigerator.

Wash the cucumber and cut into thick slices. Set aside.

Peel the lemon and cut lengthwise in half. Set aside.

Wash the basil thoroughly and roughly chop it. Set aside.

Now, combine tomato, avocado, cucumber, lemon and basil in a juicer and process until juiced.

Transfer to serving glasses and add some ice before serving.

Enjoy!

Nutrition information per serving: Kcal: 240, Protein: 3.1g, Carbs: 75.1g, Fats: 0.9g

42.   Parsnip Zucchini Juice

Ingredients:

1 cup of parsnips, chopped

1 large zucchini, seeded

1 cup of sweet potatoes, chopped

1 ginger root slice, 1-inch

2 oz of water

Preparation:

Wash the parsnips and trim off the green parts. Cut into thick slices and fill the measuring cup. Reserve the rest for some other juice.

Peel the zucchini and cut in half. Scrape out the seeds with a spoon. Cut into chunks and set aside.

Peel the sweet potato and cut into chunks. Fill the measuring cup and reserve the rest for some other juice. Set aside.

Peel the ginger root and set aside.

Now, process parsnips, zucchini, sweet potato, and ginger in a juicer.

Transfer to serving glasses and stir in the water.

Refrigerate for 10 minutes before serving.

Nutrition information per serving: Kcal: 216, Protein: 7.6g, Carbs: 61.1g, Fats: 1.5g

43.   Pomegranate Beets Juice

Ingredients:

1 cup of pomegranate seeds

1 cup of beets, trimmed and chopped

1 large lime, peeled

2 large carrots

1 large cucumber

Preparation:

Cut the top of the pomegranate fruit using a sharp knife. Slice down to each of the white membranes inside of the fruit. Pop the seeds into a measuring cup and set aside.

Wash the beets and trim off the green parts. Cut into bite-sized pieces and fill the measuring cup. Reserve the rest for some other juice.

Peel the lime and cut into lengthwise in half. Set aside.

Wash the carrot and cucumber and cut into thick slices. Set aside.

Now, process pomegranate seeds, beets, lime, carrots and cucumber in a juicer.

Transfer to serving glasses and stir in the water. Add some ice and serve!

Nutrition information per serving: Kcal: 194, Protein: 7.2g, Carbs: 57.7g, Fats: 1.9g

44. Coconut Berry Juice

Ingredients:

1 cup of blackberries

1 cup of blueberries

1 cup of strawberries

1 cup of raspberries

1 cup of cranberries

3 oz of coconut water

Preparation:

Combine blackberries, blueberries, strawberries, raspberries, and cranberries in a colander. Wash under cold running water. Cut the strawberries in half and set aside.

Now, place all berries in a juicer and process until juiced.

Transfer to serving glasses and add some ice before serving.

Enjoy!

Nutrition information per serving: Kcal: 210, Protein: 5.9g, Carbs: 75.3g, Fats: 2.5g

45.   Watermelon Mint Juice

Ingredients:

1 cup of watermelon, chopped

1 large orange, peeled

1 large peach, pitted and halved

1 large Fuji apple, cored

3 tbsp of fresh mint, chopped

Preparation:

Cut the watermelon lengthwise. For two cups, you will need about two large wedges. Peel and cut into chunks. Remove the seeds and set aside. Reserve the rest of the melon for some other juices.

Peel the orange and divide into wedges. Set aside.

Wash the peach and cut in half. Remove the pit and cut into chunks. Set aside.

Wash the apple and remove the core. Cut into bite-sized pieces and set aside.

Now, combine watermelon, orange, peach, and apple in a juicer and process until juiced.

Transfer to serving glasses and garnish with some fresh mint. Add some ice cubes before serving.

Enjoy!

Nutrition information per serving: Kcal: 269, Protein: 5.3g, Carbs: 78.5g, Fats: 1.3g

46.   Plums & Beet Juice

Ingredients:

5 large plums, pitted and halved

1 cup of purple cabbage, torn

1 whole cucumber

1 large lemon, peeled

1 cup of beets, trimmed

2 oz of water

Preparation:

Wash the plums and cut in half. Remove the pits and cut into quarters. Set aside.

Wash the cabbage thoroughly under cold running water. Drain and torn with hands.

Wash the cucumber and cut into thick slices. Set aside.

Peel the lemon and cut lengthwise in half. Set aside.

Wash the beets and trim off the green parts. Cut into bite-sized pieces and set aside.

Now, process plums, cabbage, cucumber, lemon, and beets in a juicer.

Transfer to serving glasses and add some ice before serving.

Enjoy!

Nutrition information per serving: Kcal: 243, Protein: 8.3g, Carbs: 73.6g, Fats: 1.7g

47.   Avocado Juice

Ingredients:

1 cup of avocado, sliced

3 cups of red leaf lettuce, torn

1 large orange, peeled

½ cup of pure coconut water, unsweetened

1 tsp of liquid honey

Preparation:

Peel the avocado and cut in half. Remove the pit and chop into chunks. Fill the measuring cup and reserve the rest for some other juice. Set aside.

Wash the lettuce thoroughly under cold running water. Torn with hands and set aside.

Peel the orange and divide into wedges. Set aside.

Now, combine avocado, lettuce, and orange in a juicer and process until juiced.

Transfer to serving glasses and refrigerate for 10 minutes before serving.

Enjoy!

Nutrition information per serving: Kcal: 240, Protein: 4.9g, Carbs: 25.6g, Fats: 21.7g

48.   Mixed Berry Juice

Ingredients:

1 cup of blueberries

1 cup of strawberries

1 cup of cranberries

1 cup of raspberries

1 cup of blackberries

1 small granny Smith apple

¼ cup of water

1 tsp of pure coconut sugar

2 oz of water

Preparation:

Combine all berries in a colander and wash under cold running water. Cut the strawberries in half and set aside.

Soak the berries in water for 10 minutes. Drain and set aside.

Wash the apple and remove the core. Cut into bite-sized pieces and set aside.

Now, process all berries and apple in a juicer.

Transfer to serving glasses and stir in the coconut sugar and water.

Add some ice and serve!

Nutrition information per serving: Kcal: 210, Protein: 5.7g, Carbs: 82g, Fats: 2.4g

49.   Orange Green Juice

Ingredients:

1 cup of broccoli, chopped

1 cup of Brussels sprouts, chopped

1 cup of carrots, sliced

1 cup of turnip greens, chopped

4 large oranges, peeled

1 tbsp of honey

¼ cup of pure coconut water

Preparation:

Wash the broccoli and cut into small pieces. Set aside.

Wash the Brussels sprouts and trim off the outer layers. Cut in half and set aside.

Wash the carrots and cut into thick slices. Set aside.

Wash the turnip greens thoroughly and torn with hands. Set aside.

Peel the oranges and divide into wedges. Set aside.

Now, combine broccoli, Brussels sprouts, carrots, turnip greens, and oranges in a juicer and process until juiced.

Transfer to serving glasses and stir in the honey and coconut water. Add some ice cubes before serving or refrigerate for 10 minutes.

Enjoy!

Nutrition information per serving: Kcal: 367, Protein: 14.47g, Carbs: 116g, Fats: 1.9g

50.   Fresh Apple and Cucumber Juice

Ingredients:

3 large Granny Smith apples, cored

1 large lemon, peeled

4 cups of cucumber

¼ cup of water

1 tbsp of liquid honey

Preparation:

Wash the apples and remove the core. Cut into bite-sized pieces and set aside.

Peel the lemon and cut lengthwise in half. Set aside.

Wash the cucumber and cut into thick slices. Set aside.

Now, combine apples, lemon and cucumber in a juicer and process until juiced. Transfer to serving glasses and stir in the water and liquid honey.

Garnish with some fresh mint, but this is optional.

Add few ice cubes before serving and enjoy!

Nutrition information per serving: Kcal: 327, Protein: 4.7g, Carbs: 97g, Fats: 1.5g

51.   Minty Apricot Juice

Ingredients:

5 apricots, sliced

1 large peach, sliced

1 large kiwi, peeled

A bunch of fresh spinach, chopped

1 tbsp of fresh mint, chopped

¼ cup of water

Preparation:

Wash the apricots and cut in half. Remove the pits and cut into chunks. Set aside.

Wash the peach and cut in half. Remove the pit and cut into small pieces. Set aside.

Peel the kiwi and cut lengthwise in half. Set aside.

Wash the spinach and mint under cold running water. Drain and roughly chop it. Set aside.

Now, combine apricots, peach, kiwi, spinach, and mint in a juicer and process until juiced.

Transfer to serving glasses and refrigerate before serving.

Nutrition information per serving: Kcal: 211, Protein: 2.8g, Carbs: 58.8g, Fats: 2.8g

52.   Guava Ginger Juice

Ingredients:

1 large guava, chopped

1 ginger root slice, 1-inch

4 cups of Swiss chard, torn

4 cups of fresh kale, torn

A bunch of spinach, torn

¼ cup of pure coconut water, unsweetened

1 tbsp of pure coconut sugar

Preparation:

Wash the guava and cut into chunks. Set aside.

Peel the ginger slice and set aside.

Combine Swiss chard, kale, and spinach in a colander and wash thoroughly under cold running water. Drain and torn with hands. Set aside.

Now, combine guava, ginger, Swiss chard, kale, and spinach in a juicer and process until juiced.

Transfer to serving glasses and stir in the coconut water and pure coconut sugar.

Add some ice and serve immediately.

Nutrition information per serving: Kcal: 287, Protein: 30.8g, Carbs: 80g, Fats: 6.7g

ADDITIONAL TITLES FROM THIS AUTHOR

70 Effective Meal Recipes to Prevent and Solve Being Overweight: Burn Fat Fast by Using Proper Dieting and Smart Nutrition

By

Joe Correa CSN

48 Acne Solving Meal Recipes: The Fast and Natural Path to Fixing Your Acne Problems in Less Than 10 Days!

By

Joe Correa CSN

41 Alzheimer's Preventing Meal Recipes: Reduce or Eliminate Your Alzheimer's Condition in 30 Days or Less!

By

Joe Correa CSN

70 Effective Breast Cancer Meal Recipes: Prevent and Fight Breast Cancer with Smart Nutrition and Powerful Foods

By

Joe Correa CSN

www.ingramcontent.com/pod-product-compliance
Lightning Source LLC
Chambersburg PA
CBHW030249030426
42336CB00009B/315